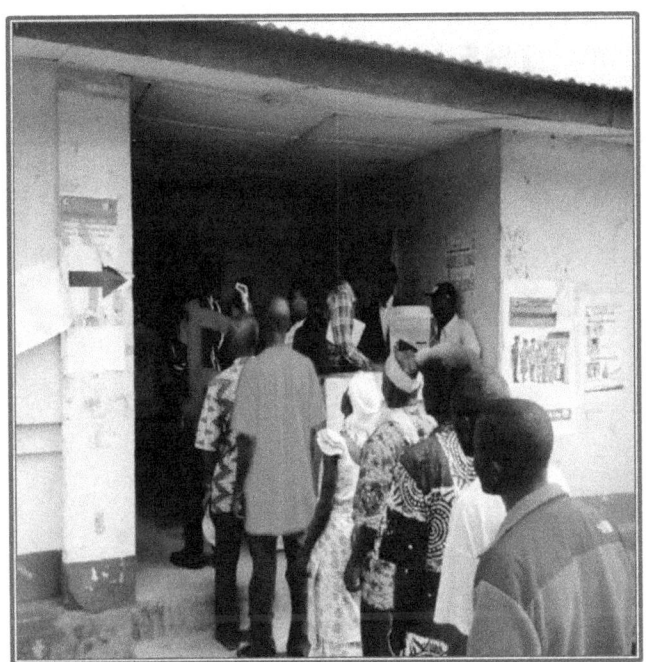

THE VILLAGE DOCTOR

BY

NWANI CHRISTIAN

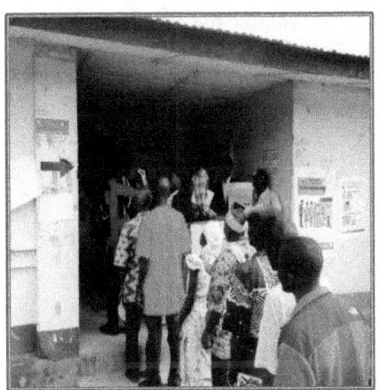

Photo used in cover is called Meeting of Chiefs.   It is located with the CDC. www.cdc.gov/vhf/ebola

Photo has been slightly modified via cropping..

https://www.flickr.com/photos/cdcglobal/15486889075/in/album-72157646018355339/

Any comments or questions can be directed to the email:

villageboy489@gmail.com

Published By:

JRB Goode Solutions, LLC
2714 Bluff Crossing
San Antonio, Texas 78244

Table of Contents

FORWARD

With the world fast developing around us it is important that all of us, not just a few should have the ability to look at other people, other ways of life and thought, with such understanding of their needs. True understanding then becomes possible, for assistance to those whose own self-help efforts are in-adequate, and the door is opened to that comfortable sense of relief and change that can lead all to enjoyable life. The strange life and disturbing environment beyond our familiar realm of experience then becomes far less strange and disturbing. To read about other people is one of the most exciting intellectual adventures in our world, thereby making us to begin to recognize a dim reflection of ourselves. It is unfortunate that in our society, the gap between the preaching and the practice seems to be almost irreconcilable. Most people who still practice what is preached never get a reward, but then were not discouraged because, they have chosen the lifestyle and the direction in which it is leading them in changing the world.

Nkemakonam Maduka is one of those who practiced what is preached. He operated a chemist shop at the Orie market in Ameyor village with integrity. The entire village and beyond depended on him for their health needs. Was he really a medical Doctor? He was not, but there was no one else whom they consulted when sick. He automatically became their village doctor. That is the irony of life. Some of the villagers called him 'Dokinta' because the pronunciation was easy for them.

The story in this book illustrates the Ameyor village life, the dedication of the village Doctor and the damages that had been done to humanity, before a true son of the soil, who resided in the United States visited the village with his advanced skill. Dr. Timothy grew tired of the health situations of the people of his roots and he became more zealous to bring about a change, learning what was required of him. His desperation and astonishing levels of effort that he took to make the life of his own people better, triggered Dr. Greg Hill, who assisted him, in pursuing the Ameyor village course of establishing a modern hospital there in the area. They achieved that great mandate and the village Doctor was eventually recognized internationally.

This book entreats and teaches a lesson to all those who are no longer socially conscious, to those who have unwittingly abandoned their own roots everywhere in the world. It appeals and disturbs just enough, that maybe, just maybe, someone might awaken from their sleep, and truly see the world around them and its needs. And then find a way to help.

For All African Aid Donors

ACKNOWLEDGEMENTS

I am grateful to my great friend, James Regan for shouldering the huge burden in editing and publishing my first book "The Crys of the Ambitious Village Boy" at no cost. He has done it again in this particular book despite his tight schedule, to buttress his rare altruistic attitude. May God bless him all the more.

I specially thank Thomas Onyiaodike's family, Raphael Ogbodo Nwani, Ugwu Okorie and my entire family for all the powerful roles they have played in my life.

I gratefully acknowledge my august audience across the globe.

Editor's Note

Upon reading this work and having the opportunity to edit this, I was moved by the altruistic nature of this particular person, The Village Doctor. I was captivated by the Village Doctor's commitment and devotion to his local people. I was further surprised by the author's elucidation of the many local customs of the area and how they go about things. What moved me the most after I had completely read it was finding out that it was primarily fiction!

This author demonstrates his uncanny ability to weave fiction as truth. But then again, I think fiction being used as a writing vehicle allows more inward truth to be revealed many times over when compared to the story being told as is. Fiction itself has the unique ability to engross, captivate and eventually inspire the reader. In this case I believe the reader here is being inspired to take action. I will allow you to find out for yourself just how intriguing this message really is and what action specifically you are being inspired and asked to do.

James Regan

1

The Ameyor Village

The Ameyor Village was one of the most blasé places in Eastern Nigeria. Lying flat exactly in Nkanu Land, it presented the dark and lowering image of a region where huge trees rose a hundred feet. It was a place of unexpected silence, not the familiar noisy jungle, with its incessant insect buzzing and bird screeching. The immensity of the woodland seemed to muffle the noise. The mold of dead leaves covering the ground absorbed footfalls and the general gloom, a gloom where the sunlight failed to penetrate the dense foliage creating thus a somber, sepulchral quality. The people biologically and naturally had adapted to the village, and lived in a close and cheerful symbiotic relationship to it. They regarded it as their close ally, provider, and refuge. If taken away from it, serious lassitude could set in. Movement between the immense tree trunks was easy enough for a small person, and nimble one far easier. Edible fruits, and plants, as well as wild animals, could sustain skilled and active villagers. Above all, the village offered sanctuary. One still wonders the fearsome image that discouraged the white explorers from bringing civilization to the people of the area centuries ago. They raised *crops, possessed domestic animals and a dog that must have a wooden* bell hung around its neck while hunting. The search for water was the starkest challenge that the villagers must meet during the dry season. They travelled miles to fetch. If a sequence of water supplies fails, the villagers are faced with disaster. As a precaution, the water carrier may carry water for a long journey in a basin or bucket with twigs floating in it to prevent splashing. In the begging, the river itself was the only highway through the region. Near the water was heard the evening chorus frogs or, at dawn. But for most of the day there was nothing but the sudden harsh croak of the hornbill to punctuate the stillness.

As gatherers of vegetable products and small insects, the women need little more than a simple digging stick, to turn up underground roots and burrowing grubs, and the characteristic shallow bowl in which to carry their harvest. Some of them were used as scoops when winnowing the chaff from wild-grass grains, or as a mixing bowl when preparing food, or even still, as water carriers when moving from one water hole to the next during the rainy season. To establish camp in the farm was not a simplicity. In areas, where frequent rainfall is expected, the villagers preferred to build huts out of local materials; bark lean-tos, grass houses, or bark-strip sheds that propped up out of the flood water.

The gathering of wild foods in the bush was done mostly by the women, though the art was not strictly confined to them, as there were men here and there who gave their time to it. They searched for edible mushrooms and fungi, sweet root, nuts, and berries. These were collected and placed in baskets. Women and girls would go gathering woods, forest products, as the Ameyor village was a bountiful provider. The collecting of wild products was a haphazard but successful operation. The women gleaned food and other necessities from the jungle, as they passed through on their way to the hunting or farm lands. They had the ability to spot things while moving at a fast pace. They were never idle. At the same time, there were the traditional rendezvous for the township. Women operating at the market, permitted them to obtain the village things; especially palm oil, enabling them too, to establish a cash base.

Honey gathering, because it involved climbing the tree or cutting it down, was usually done by the men. The honey was usually found high up in the rotten branches, or low holes of some of the trees. The entrance to the hive was widened with a few strokes of an ax. A leaf tube containing smoldering embers was poked into the hole, and the person puffs through the tube until the clouds of smoke drive away the bees. Then the collector puts his arm, scoops out handfuls of honey, and drops them in the basin. From this they had a way of making money. Even the poorest grade of honey, clouded with dirt and broken bark, was salvaged.

Most of the villagers had a complex internal affinity by patrilineal, but each nuclear family living in its own house, had lesser responsibility. Young children and youths formed associations of their own age groups, each group behaving and learning what was required of them till they die. Unnecessary noise, needless destruction of plants, uncouth behavior – all were considered to be insulting to the village. Being excellent linguistics, they had learned the several dialects necessary to communicate with communities in various parts of the region.

Here, the women were the chief potters and calabash makers. It was the lower class for whom vessels were required, and they could not afford to purchase them from professional potters, but made them for their households, whatever pots they required. There can be little doubt that these type of pots, and indeed the art of making them, had filtered into Ezilo, Izii and other communities in the Ebonyi State. The work they produced there was a higher standard of style and workmanship than in the humbler class. All pottery was made by hand, and no attempt has been made, to use any kind of wheel for the cylindrical pots. Still, the shapes were wonderfully true and the curves of some of the water storing pots were beautifully formed. As the clay is seldom well worked or prepared and the pots were never thoroughly burned, the vessels became brittle, and unless frequently re-dried in the sun or over a fire, they were liable to break when carried or lifted. The tools used were of a very local character. For example, a piece of a gourd formed a resting platform for the base of the pot, while the sides were being built up, and another small piece was used as a trowel until the whole pot was completed. Such pots were kept some days, and when fairly hard were exposed to the sun until quite dry. They were then heaped together, covered with grass and reeds and were set on fire, kept there until they were quite hard. The potter thus can obtain a fine black or brown polish, which he burns on, which would last the life-time of the pot.

Basketry was carried on by both children and adult men, in some places almost entirely by the children, the men folk making only the stronger and larger mat-baskets for drying farm produce. The finer basket-work was done by them, who prepared certain grasses and the fronds of palm leaves and aloes for their work.

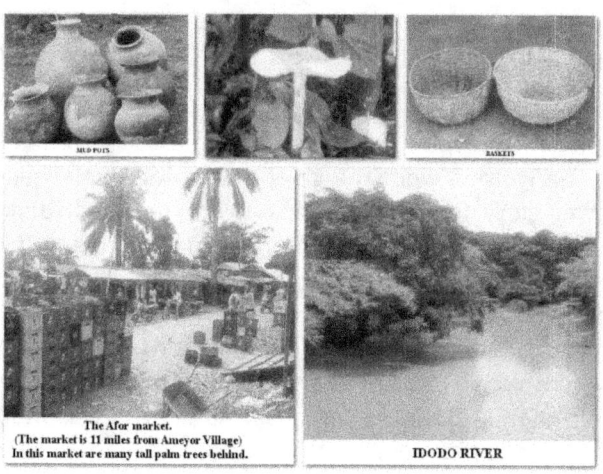

The Afor market.
(The market is 11 miles from Ameyor Village)
In this market are many tall palm trees behind.

IDODO RIVER

The people of this region enjoyed good health and were quite free from serious illnesses as other tribes in Africa, until few years ago when science and technology began to play both positive and negative roles in people's lives. The villagers had many strange ideas as to what was the cause of illness, so that, when they had anything wrong with them, they would be subjected to a great amount of doctoring; herbs, leaves, barks, and shrubs. The medicine man or woman (dibia) is called in or visited, not only to cure the patient, but also to decide whether the sickness was caused by magic, and, if so, to discover who has been at work and why. As a cure he may order the patient to drink an infusion of herbs, or he may advise blistering. At other times he ordered the application of a plaster of herbs.

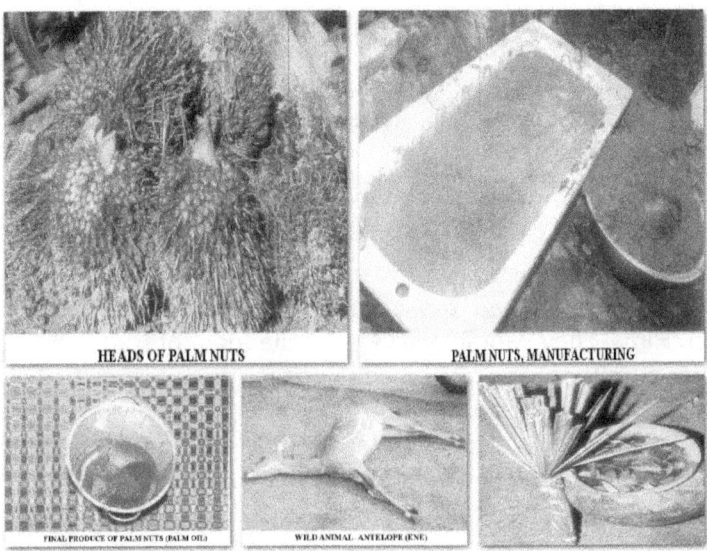

HEADS OF PALM NUTS   PALM NUTS, MANUFACTURING

FINAL PRODUCE OF PALM NUTS (PALM OIL)   WILD ANIMAL ANTELOPE (ENE)

When a man is said to be under the influence of magic or charm, it was the duty of the relatives to do what they could to have the person freed, and they subjected the person to a man who professes to have the necessary knowledge and power. Should he pronounce the illness to be of a particular spirit (Ogbanje) he has to discover whether it was a spirit belonging to the clan or some hostile spirit from another clan that was at work. A spirit belonging to the family may give trouble because the family as a whole had transgressed in some way or some member of it had committed an immoral act which the spirit resents. Spirits were ever watching over the affairs of the clan to keep its members from straying from the right path. On the other hand, spirits from other clans may come with evil intent, causing illness or possibly death. Those had to be captured and destroyed; but the spirit of a member of the clan has to be persuaded to forgive the offence and come out of the patient and to accomplish this, the relatives would give it large presents for sacrifices. Medicine men or women, endowed with strong supernatural powers, interceded with the spiritual world, for good or evil, on behalf of individuals or a group. Despite their stately notions of personal etiquette, the villagers observed very few of those rituals often associated with life's major turning points. For this purpose, there was in every home a shrine before which food, kolanut and chicken are placed for the gods annually especially during the iriaju festival.

They acknowledged the existence of a creator but they didn't worship Him. They worshiped Ani – the god of the land. Certain servants (Umunna) became their priest, and there had been a succession of these mediums from that time to this. This god was only appealed to on special occasions; he was called upon during war, when there was any trouble among the people or for success in venture. Local amulets were worn by men and some women at all times, for everyone wore a special charm, as protection against any complaint to which he, or she, is particularly subjected to; but the god and custom of the land were kept before the minds of the people. Large sums were paid for a good fetish to be made by the native doctor of one of the deities.

Thunder and lightning (egbigwe) were attributed to the movements of one and the manifestation of another. Thus, when any calamity happened, and either men or trees were struck by lightning and the trees would block the roads, a ritual must be made with nturu to the gods before the rest of trees or dead body can be taken away from the place where they had been struck down. The nturu was usually in possession of the Umuna or clan whose duty was to officiate in the village shrine.

Should a rich man organize a burial ceremony in honor of his late mother or father, a hunt was organized, in which seven to twenty men took part. A few men followed the track of an animal and discovered its haunts so that, when other hunters arrived, they could tell them. The haunts-men made a wide ring and advanced, beating down the grass, ever narrowing their circle until they came upon the animal. It was seldom, that any man was wounded in such a hunt. The hunts men returned singing with double barrel guns as they marched through the compound, where the funeral ceremony was being held, and every other event would stop performing, until certain gun shots were heard in a particular target.

To a visitor from an enlightened society the most immediate striking feature of the village life, even in the most local form, was its astonishing ability to appreciate visitors, which included a certain respect for manners and not an affront. They were naturally chummy.

There was a good deal of evidence showing that the work of the Christian missionaries, who began to have a real effect in Amayor village many years ago, was by no means the first influence on the Ameyor religious beliefs. Nothing could have been culturally challenging than the Christian mission's ascendance, with its new rules for everything; from circumcision to coffin and into the spirit world beyond. They negotiated with the people in charge, preached to the common people, taught new ways of life but failed to establish hospitals and schools, as they did in many other communities. Yet, as their vocation demanded, the missionaries were also concerned in saving souls. Their dedication was beyond question. Their very presence divided the villager's religious belief. Some were converted while others remained with the crude African tradition. That's how, we Christians over here, undermined the foundation of our own cultures – although we did not regret it, because, we feel the presence of the Heavenly Host everyday in our lives.

However, it was in this particular village, that Nkemakonam Maduka, was generally known as the village Doctor. He was the one who introduced the new system of heterodox medicine to the people, while he operated his chemist shop at the Orie Market. He was well specialized and strongly informed about current practice in the township, where he used to attend seminars, workshops and other health programs. He operated his chemist shop for many years in the city before he moved down to the village. The man himself was slender in build; he had thin limbs, chocolate-dark skin, and delicately

17

formed hands and feet. His face bore a vaguely familiar, faintly West African cast, and his nose had pronounced bulbous tips. For ten years he labored as a village Doctor of the Ameyor natives and beyond, helping them to focus attention on their health problems.

2

At the Chemist Shop

He was still mixing drugs for the baby suffering from pneumonia when the hag sped passed the queue, and trotted right into the chemist's shop. The village Doctor could not ignore her:

"Hay! Why are you standing here? Join the Queue." He instructed.

"Dokinta, my son is badly wounded, blood is pouring off from his head! He is in front of your shop".

"Okay! Go back! I will soon come and treat him".

The villagers on the queue started murmuring over the woman's haste in rushing to the Doctor without first joining the queue. Many of them had stood there for 15 minutes, others had stayed for 30 minutes or more waiting for the village Doctor to mix drugs for them. The village Doctor himself, was not very comfortable sitting down for long hours, attending to the people. Sweat was pouring off of him, because the two windows were not enough in providing adequate ventilation. His dogged hands were very busy, as he opened the poured drugs and closed the drug carns. He could not make much use of the hand fan in front of him because of his desperately busy hands. The spoon and stainless plate with which he mixed these drugs had suffered – white chalk colored them. As he was still working hard to contain the pressure placed on him from his villager customers, the tattered man spoke up.

"Dokinta! I am still waiting for you to inject me."

"Is it time?"

Yes! You said 5 O' clock. It's 5 p.m. already!"

"Okay! Hold on, I will attend to you soon."

The tattered man walked back to his seat in frustration, and sat sluggishly on the bench again in the corridor very close to the hag. The queue kept growing even as others left the shop with their own drugs.

After a couple of minutes, the village Doctor rose with the hand fan on his left hand fanning himself. He took hold of the treatment box and was about to make his way out of the shop when the average fair man shouted!

"Doctor! I am dying! Do not allow me to defecate in your shop."

"What's wrong with you?"

"Loose bowel. I have been defecating uncontrollably since yesterday. The leaves I have been chewing I have now abruptly refused, to stop the stomach problem."

The Doctor dropped the treatment box, picked a card of Flagyl (400mg) and cut it into two. He gave it to the man and asked him to take two tablets immediately. The man fetched water with a plastic cup, from the blue plastic bucket in the shop, and drank without delay. The good traditional drug money was paid, and he went-back home with the remaining drugs. The village Doctor appealed to the villagers to wait for him so that he could attend to an emergency case. He took hold of the box again and gradually made his way towards the young man in pool of blood. When he saw him, he exclaimed!

"Ah! Ah! What happen to you?"

"I fell from the mangoes tree when I was plucking the ripped mangoes, my head smashed on the sharp stone when I landed."

"Sorry! Be still"

He had already opened the box and brought the wool, spirit, ink and others and as he cleaned the wound, the young boy screamed painfully. Her mother held his hands so much so to stop him from distorting the good treatment. The Doctor kept pouring liquids and cleaning them under the watchful eyes of the hag and spectators from the village market. The wound was well cleaned and sealed up. He instructed him sternly not to bathe the affected part and that he should be careful while lying down so much so to protect the bandage. He also asked them to return in seven days. They thanked him and went back home.

No sooner had the Doctor finished the treatment, that pressure was mounted on him again and again. The Queue kept growing as those who had come to patronize his drugs, and had joined through numerous footsteps. An angry tattered man was invited for his infection. He was taken inside to an alternate tiny blue corner of the shop. The village Doctor gave him a proportional tetanus injection to curtail the stiffness in his body system. The tattered man screamed angrily as the Doctor used the wool and massaged the injection spot. The village Doctor spoke to him after the message:

"Nails are dangerous, come again by tomorrow at 5 p.m. for another tetanus injection. Be careful with your working tools so that, you won't step on another nail."

"Okay! Thank you very much. Let me be on my way." The tattered man struggled, staggered and trotted out. A nursing mother then spoke up from behind;

"Dokinta! My son is alone in the house down with measles. He is 7 months; please give me drugs for him."

Another nursing mother who was tetchy responded:

"You have just come to the shop now, and you are shouting to the Doctor to attend to you, but we have been here for a long time without complaining, neither shouting. Dokinta; don't mind her. I need diarrhea drug for my kid. She is six months."

The women retorted and they began to quarrel, they called each other all sorts of names in abuse. Their breasts kept jumping as they got ready to fight; none of them wore a bra. The tetchy woman stretched her hand to hit her, when the voice of the Doctor was heard:

"Madam! Take your diarrhea drug. You too, take your measles drugs. You mothers should give them as prescribed." All these whiles, that they were quarreling, the Doctor was busy mixing drugs for them hence peace was eventually restored in the shop corridor. He collected his money from them; and the measles woman bade him au revoir.

At 7 p.m. Ezeobu was crying along the village road bare footed, heading to the chemist shop, inside his hand were onions, part of which he chewed along the way. Ezeobu got to the shop lamenting of the exquisite pain of a bite. He kept raising his voice in anguish. The Doctor was still busy attending to those in the queue. Ezeobu was well known by him.

He asked,

"Ezeobu what happen to you?"

"A scorpion has mercilessly bitten me where I was covering pieces of palm nuts. I have already taken two heads of onions finely. This one is the third."

"Do you think that chewing these onions will relieve the pain?"

"I think so. That's what people use and the pain would stop, but mine seems to be different" The Doctor smiled and responded;

"You need to wait for 7 minutes; I'm already mixing drugs for those who came before you. First come, first serve, is the law of this shop,"

"Dokinta! It is too painful to wait on; the brown scorpion targeted me wrongly."

"Ezeobu! Did you kill the scorpion, or you allowed it to escape?"

"I was able to kill it. I believe by now fire has consumed it, I put it in the fire,"

"Okay. I'm coming."

How Ezeobu was sobbing uncontrollably, made everyone in the chemist shop understand that the scorpion bite was a very excruciating kind of pain. So, the village Doctor when he was done with the customer on desk walked him into the injection corner and injected him. He asked him to remain for him to know how he would fare with the injection. Ezeobu shambled to the corridor and the Doctor went ahead attending to the numerous customers. In a couple of minutes, Ezeobu uttered to the Doctor!

"The bite no longer pains me."

"Good! Be mindful of insects and rodents in your farm work".

"Okay! Please permit me to pay by tomorrow. The acute pain made me to forget money and my slippers at home."

"You can go. Pay up by tomorrow so that I won't have to close this shop." Ezeobu accepted, because he knew that if money doesn't flow into the shop, the village Doctor cannot serve them better. The village Doctor was indeed merciful. Ezeobu left.

At 7:30 p.m., a group of people were moaning miserably coming towards the chemist shop. The village Doctor was very busy mixing drugs and pretended to be deaf to the loud cries. It mostly tinkled the ears when the crowd stopped in front of his ever busy shop, amidst tears. A tall huge man was lowered in flat on the plank, as white foam was gushing out of his mouth. The man could not raise his hand, feet neither talked. He needed urgent medical attention. The wife flailed around in a gushed emotion. The doctor rose in a burning zeal to save the man. As he walked to the corridor, his box scratched the big blue burning lamp and it fell. The glass broke and the light went out. The corridor was sounding with the crowd, including spectators and the sick ones. He bent low, picked the lamp up and went back to the shop to replace it. A woman helped, and picked up the broken pieces. He returned with the lamp burning with new flames and queried:

"What is wrong with Onochie?"

"I don't know. I went to the back yard to pack cloths, when I returned, I found him in this situation." The wife answered.

"Okay! Let me check his B.P."

"B.P? What is B.P?"

"Madam! B.P. is blood pressure."

"Blood pressure? Dokinta! Please treat my husband, he is at the point of death and you are here standing, talking about blood pressure. My husband has a lot of blood inside him."

"Madam! Allow me to do my work now that Mr. Onochie is still breathing."

"I beg of you. Do your work and save my husband."

The village Doctor was already checking Mr. Onochie's B.P., the blood pressure read low. He quickened his pace into the shop and took hold of a tiny bottle, and took few paces back and gave him an injection. Again, he checked the sugar level and it was very low. He rushed and picked another small bottle in a bucket of water, and returned quickly. He used the syringe and drew a proportional milligram amount, which he injected into Mr. Onochie's muscles. There were harsh whispers of another new terminal emergency, but the village Doctor remained focused treating Mr. Onochie. He injected two more drugs and urged the family to monitor him. So, he stood up and looked at the new case. It was a miserably pale man. He asked the man's family;

"What's wrong with him?"

"I don't really know. He keeps fainting." The answer was produced by the man's wife.

"Okay! Go and buy a bottle of sprite for him."

"I have no money, Dokinta."

The village Doctor provided money, and the woman rushed to the nearby store, she bought a bottle of sprite and ran back. She extended it to the husband and he quickly collected it from her. The speed, at which he gulped down the sprite, amazed the village Doctor. He provided another amount of money to buy food from the nearby restaurant, a plate of jollof rice was quickly bought, and carried to him, and the man ate with indecent haste. The village Doctor shook his head and scratched it. He trotted into his shop and sat down. It was succinctly obvious that Mr. Obiakor was starving. Hunger fainted him. The village Doctor called Mrs. Obiakor into the shop and as he was extending money to her urged;

"Go and buy food for the family. If your husband faints again, do not hesitate in bringing him."

"Thank you Dokinta! It's as if you know, my husband has not eaten for three days, there is no food in the house. He fainted where he was cultivating with his hoe at the farm."

"Okay! He should not be cultivating while on empty stomach". She collected the money and went into the shops to buy food stuff. When she returned to pick her husband, Mr. Onochie gave a violent sneeze and opened his eyes. The spectators were amazed and the village Doctor stood in awe and wondered. Mr. Onochie looked at his wife, children and all those gathered in the thick dark, gazing at him. He became confused and rose from the plank angrily. He threw two awful questions immediately:

"Why am I here? Why is everyone gazing at me steadily?" He was deeply embarrassed by their prying eyes, enough to wonder how he knew they were looking at him for a long time to see if he could show signs of being alive. Mrs. Onochie became exhilarated by the question and she quickly answered.

"Nnanyi! Sickness brought us here. Thanks to God, you are able to talk to me again."

Mr. Onochie became speechless, they supported him and he sat down on the bench to get a better view of all those who were concerned about him; both men and women hugged him. Low blood pressure and low sugar level could be dangerous, when not closely monitored. The village Doctor spoke up from his chair inside the shop:

"Mr. Onochie! I am very happy that you made it. Be careful with what you eat. I will place you on daily medication because your blood sugar level is threatening your life span. I shall come to your house by tomorrow morning to check up your B.P and sugar level. I will also come with pamphlet menu for people as you. I believe your wife will adhere to the dietary."

"Dokinta! Tell him ooh! He drinks a lot of palm wine every day. He doesn't know he is no longer a youth." Mrs. Onochie submitted.

"As I have said, I will be in your house by tomorrow morning, we shall discuss further upon my arrival. Take this drugs, ensure, he takes them before bed."

"Thank you very much indeed."

Mrs. Onochie received the drugs and they went off happily. Therefore, the discharge of Mr. Obiakor and Onochie dismissed the crowd at the chemist shop. Only three people remained there to get medical attention. The villagers knew quite well, the village Doctor closes his shop at 9.00 p.m. every day, and they came to the shop within the hour, but, the humble Doctor had never abandoned any emergency while working to beat the clock.

The village Doctor thought that he was done with the day's emergency cases, but he did not know that more still awaited him. A boy ran to him with blood flowing down the legs from his left thigh. The boy was a basket maker. He was making a basket when a thorn of the palm frond pierced through the huge deposit of flesh. As he was drawing the thorn out of the thigh, it broke; this made him to run as fast as his legs could carry him unto the Doctor. So, the ever willing Doctor gave him an injection for pain reliefs before he proceeded with the minor operation. The tiny thorn was carefully removed and he stitched the wound and bandaged it. He warned him not to continue basket making until the stitches are removed. The boy of 12 agreed, and as he was about to leave, a man and a woman appeared on the corridor.

However, the woman was being held by her husband, one of her legs was up as she tottered. Her instep was blood. She was restless and lines of worry were deeply etched across her paused lips.

"What happen to your wife?" the Doctor Queried.

"A broken bottle pierced her when she marched on it unawares. It seems a piece of it is still in the leg based on the sensation which reflects in her moan." The village Doctor bent low and began to treat her. Blood kept dripping out as the village Doctor cleaned the wound. He injected the woman to control the pain and flow of blood, after which, he continued cleaning and searching, until he discovered a shard. She wailed with pain as he was removing it. He eventually succeeded in removing the shard. He treated the wound and sealed it with a bandage. The woman was a bit relieved of the bearing of long pain. The painstaking attention of the village Doctor to every detail of the cases that were brought to him, saved many lives. They were grateful to the Doctor, and the husband paid a certain amount. The man was glad to see her wife feel better and they went back home.

The village Doctor quickly closed his shop. He rode his bicycle to the house of Mrs. Odinaka, who was suffering from chicken pox by 9:00 p.m. The disease had already spread rapidly over her body, before the village Doctor was consulted. She used to do 'self-medication', yet it had failed her. The medication she fondly used was carm wood, which she rubbed on her body every night but when the village Doctor started treating her, there was an improvement. It became a routine of the Doctor to attend to her morning and night every day. Mrs. Odinaka had suffered seclusion; she was excluded from the public due to the high density of the infections disease on her body. On that day, the village Doctor encouraged her and gave her the normal dosage of the day's injection.

At last, the day's tedious work was over. He climbed the bicycle and headed home to refreshing up and to begin again by tomorrow. He treated the villagers genuinely and benignly – a demonstration of genuine concern in making the village salubrious.

3

Absent

At 4:00 p.m., the villagers had begun to queue up towards the chemist shop. They were all waiting patiently for the arrival of the village Doctor to attend to them as usual. Under-aged children were crying out, here and there, helplessly. Some of them were backed by their mothers while others were carried with hands. Their mothers tried to breast feed them but they rejected the good offer. Many of the villagers started going to the village Doctor's residence for him to attend to them there. Those villagers were disappointed as well because he was not at home either, so they turned back to the shop in desperation. Some of them sat on the bare floor, others sat on the available bench while others stood up waiting. Some were chatting slowly, some were angry, and some were murmuring. An old man could not bear the Doctor's absence; he fainted and died at the spot. He was suffering from cirrhosis. The crowd roared with pain and they all wept, fear grieved them because they did not know who was next to fall among them. Concerned villagers took the dead body home. The old man would have not died if the village Doctor had been on duty. Despite the fact that a man had lost his life, the villagers still kept coming to see if they themselves could get medical attention. The atmosphere was quite tense, as there was no news about the village Doctor's whereabouts. What mental states that could be seen around the chemist shop were desperation, confusion, commotion, distress, disappointment, and helplessness among the villagers. Yes! They felt the village Doctor's absence because; there was no one else in his stead.

The village Doctor in his tireless effort to serve the village better went to the Enugu city to buy more drugs, but something happened to him, he fainted suddenly at the drug market. Hence the drug distributor and three meek people rushed him to the nearest city's hospital for immediate treatment. This marred his plans to return to the village. He stayed in the hospital all through the day and night, unconscious. He woke eventually the following morning becoming vaguely conscious that he was in a hospital and being watched by a nurse. For this reason, he threw out a terrible question to her.

"How did I come in here?" The nurse calmed him and told him the story. He was feeble and could not say many words. The drug distributor visited later in the day and offset some bills in his behalf. They discussed briefly and he went back. The village Doctor was gradually having a palpable sense of relief.

It struck His Royal Majesty forcibly how the village man died in front of the chemist shop. He became anxious to know about the cause of the village Doctor's absence. Through ardent curiosity, the council of elders got wind that the village doctor was hospitalized. The elders were concerned and they had an inquisitive mind about their indigenes. Moping around won't help the villagers! Therefore, the village leader and his entourage travelled to the city to see the true son of the soil. They located the city's hospital and ward. The receptionist took them to the room where the village Doctor laid on the hospital bed on drip; seeing them in the flesh gladdened his heart. He was a man of true worth and very important to the people of the area. They exchanged greetings and he was consoled, but he was surprised at how quickly they visited him and he was very happy. The dutiful nurse alerted the medical Doctor in-charge of the case about the presence of the Royal Majesty in the hospital. He came quickly to pay homage. It was during their discussion that one of the vocal entourage uttered:

"Doctor Sir! People in the village are dying away because of your patient's absence. Discharge him." The medical Doctor laughed at such an unprofessional statement, but he responded:

"This man lying here is suffering a stress-related illness. What does he do in the village?"

"He is the village Dokinta!"

"Him! The village Doctor?"

The entourage nodded in agreement. The medical Doctor stole a look of mute on the village Doctor.

"Well, he shall recover soon and will be discharged."

His Royal Majesty thanked the medical Doctor. He appealed to him to handle him with great care because the village Doctor is 'one men' and not one man; the medical Doctor did not harden his heart. He promised to discharge his duty with all sense of responsibility as a professional expertise. He left. The village Doctor and his visitors chatted briefly, he was still very weak but appreciative of their presence. Those things they bought for him were given to him. He promised to return soon to the village. They went back home safely where they informed others about the village Doctor's situation. The villagers had pity and felt sorry for him.

In the village, there were many deaths of recent, a man who had a seizure disease died. He was at the fireside warming himself after the heavy down pour when the sickness violently attacked him. It threw him into the flames and the fire burned all over him. There were other scares and sores being treated by the village Doctor. Being that the village Doctor was not in town; the family went into the bush and cut some healing leaves. The leaves were vigorously squeezed and its liquids were poured on the wounds. It was too painful for the man who had the seizures; he gave up after two days of the fire incident.

Mr. Onochie, who was suffering from low sugar and low B.P. died as well. Insulin was not given to him when necessary. The death toll in the village, frightened many, two children died of measles. In all, seven people had kicked the bucket within a week of the village Doctor's absence including two pregnant women. He didn't plan his absence and should have given instructions to many. It is a lesson to us all.

The village Doctor was later discharged from the hospital having fully recovered from the sudden illness. He had a healthy discussion with the medical Doctor. During their discussion, the medical Doctor made him aware he dropped suddenly in fatigue and should visit periodically for bed rest. He thanked him for his great care over him and he also briefly interacted with the dutiful nurse before he went back to the drug market to meet the distributor. When he got there, he greatly appreciated him for his prompt action in taking him to the hospital and his financial support. The drug distributor was very happy for his presence. The village Doctor really lost a lot of his belongings during the incident, but those things were like a sacrifice to him. Having spent a lot of money, he bought some drugs on credit. The drug distributor accompanied him to the mass transit and he joined the bus. He arrived to the village safety.

However, the news about the village Doctor's home coming spread rapidly, crowd gathered. They welcomed him with open arms. Yes they missed him. They did not conceal their joy at his speedy recovery and in seeing him at his usual place. He was not like those who never get back when attacked by ailment. The prayers they made for him were greatly answered by Heaven. They made him aware of the number of people that died in his absence, for this reason, they would no longer take him nor his medical advice for granted. He was struck by the incongruity of the death rate in his absence, as an indefatigable promoter of health services; he opened his shop and attended to the numerous customers who trooped out in mass, and lined up to patronize his drugs. One of the indigenes who lived in town advised him to check if there were any expired drugs and remove them. The perfectly understandable village Doctor nodded. He was often separated from any attitudes or drugs that could cost a life.

The council of elders unanimously decided to honor the village Doctor with a chieftaincy title in appreciation of his great efforts in serving the people. On that Nkwor market day, they all gathered at the village square to participate in a complete ceremony. He was dressed in the formal chieftaincy attire and cap, Ofor Igbo was given which should protect him from all danger – they believed. The villagers danced, danced and danced, the village Doctor danced too. The title of his name became 'Onye aya na nwanne ya! It coincided with his way of life. He appreciated the council of elders for giving him the recognition and encouragement. He also promised to use his experiences wisely and gain more valuable experiences through research and be in association with specialists. They all lavished a lot of time making merry at the village square. The council of elders had the villagers in the palm and the villagers had been loyal thereby, the village was accommodating to all.

4

The Palm Wine Tapper's Case

The village palm wine tappers were just as industrious as any of the other groups of people who worked in differing professions. Some of these professional wine tappers had 20-30 palm trees that they climbed daily. Every morning, they tapped the natural palm wine and poured it in a calabash or in a half gallon, which had been tied firmly to their waist. They would then peel away the hard substances that might make the natural wine taste unpleasant. After that, they retied the gallon back to themselves before climbing down carefully. The palm wine which they brought down was poured into gallons tied across the bicycle career (for those who had bicycles). When they were done tapping, they would go home to prepare the wine for the public. At home, all the natural wine tapped, was poured into a well refined mud pot and then mixed with water.

Palm wine is one of the strongest natural wines on earth hence a proportional amount of water was added to it to water it down. Therefore, when the mixing up of the wine was done, pure silk used as a sieving material would be placed over the funnel before the wine could be poured into the gallons again. Gallons were used in the selling of the palm wines and the silk would prevent any unwanted materials from gaining entrance into the prepared wine. When these processes were achieved, the gallons of wine would be kept in the sunlight for a few minutes to settle. At this juncture, the palm wine tapper would prepare for market. When he was done preparing, he would move them there to sell. Sometimes the wine sold quickly and at higher prices, that's when he would say that the market is good! When the market was bad, the wine sold at very minimal amounts and the palm wine tapper stayed for long hours awaiting patronage.

It is worthy of note that the palm wine tappers had to climb the palm trees, three times a day to remove the foams and substances on the flowering tree to produce the wine and avoid it from becoming

34

acidulous. Failure of the palm wine tapper to climb the palm tree twice again after initially tapping in the mornings, would surely make the wine have an unpleasant taste and quite hard to drink. This might result in giving him a bad reputation as a palm wine tapper and thus he could lose a lot of sales. They climbed the palm trees with a noose (agbu), a small padded knife girded around the waste, and a cutlass when necessary. Most of the palm wine tappers had bicycles for easy access to the places where the palm trees were located. The palm trees could be found at people's homes and farms in Africa. The palm wine tappers paid a certain amount to the palm tree owners and offered them wine freely once per annum. These ever busy and hard-working palm wine tappers used to be up from bed as early as 3:00 a.m. in order to enable them to finish tapping on time and then go to the market. Torches or owa, which they tied across their foreheads, provided the helpful light when shined on steadily. The villagers liked palm wine and they even went so far as booking it beforehand on occasion.

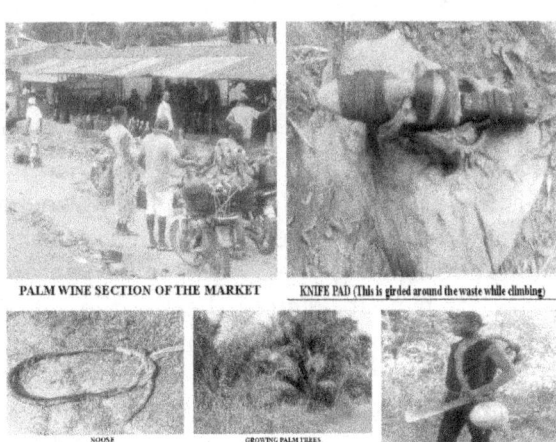

PALM WINE SECTION OF THE MARKET   KNIFE PAD (This is girded around the waste while climbing)

NOOSE   GROWING PALM TREES

Consequently this was the profession of Mr. Nworie Edeani in the village. The man cherished the good life he had, hence he was not in the habit of going to the farm when he returned from selling his palm wines. He looked strong and healthy and had a way of pushing himself while riding the bicycle in sheer joy of being alive. He was very jovial, chirpy and chummy and a man of few words. His tall dark wife was in-charge of the farm. One of the things he liked most was oyena. Oyena was a well garnished meat that was hawked at the market by a lone man. Mr. Nworie used to buy them to quench some serious concerns. He clung to the belief that life was best enjoyed with a clear mind and not a wounded heart. However, palm wine aided in entangling it.

Mr. Nworie's misery began on Thursday night when his leg slipped off from the marked points that was used for footing on the palm tree, while climbing down. He fell down from the tall palm tree and both of his legs were fractured. His agonized cries went on for long hours and were not heard by those on earth, neither did the Heavens intervene. He continued to moan miserably and helplessly until another wine tapper in a far distance overheard his expression of severe pain. Without any delay, the palm wine tapper came down from the palm tree and made his way towards Mr. Nworie. When Mr. Nworie noticed a man with torch light coming towards him, he waited in the agony of suspense. The palm wine tapper walked at close range, noticed him and groaned in anguish. He groped for Mr. Nworie's knife, found it and kept it separately. He made an attempt to lift him, but he was too heavy for him. In anguish, he ran through the village road raising a war cry. The war cry would draw the attention of the villagers quickly. So, the villagers heard him and knew that there was danger in the land. The brave villagers gathered, with the different weapons that were available to them and also brought torch lights. He took them to where Mr. Nworie lied down in lamentation and devastation. They all cried out with rage. A long door was quickly provided and Mr. Nworie was carefully transferred onto it. The able-bodied young men took him home. His family was deeply horrified by the accident and they cried out in disapproval. Their tears and wails woke those who had gone to bed hence many villagers rushed to the compound in symbolized sympathy. Five young boys were immediately sent out to summon the village Doctor, though they knew he was not an osteopath. He was summoned to take care of the bruises and perhaps administer some drugs for pain relief. The news of the accident spread slowly across the village that night. The village Doctor had already heard it said among the women. He was at home resting from the day's tiresome job.

When the five young men arrived, there was a knock on the door and the village Doctor quickly opened. They greeted him before the shortest young man broke the ugly news to him. He was exhausted but he was second to none in the village. He went inside, stayed briefly and carried the treatment box. Yes! He joined them in thick darkness. There were torch lights and lamps in Mr. Nworie's compound when they arrived. The village Doctor's presence heightened the people's emotions. He went inside the room where Mr. Nworie was dumped and languishing in great pain. He quietened the room and then began the effective treatment. The crowd outside was causing commotion but the village Doctor did not concern himself with the details as he kept himself busy. Therefore, some of the villagers went home after the treatment while others slept there in solidarity. Mr. Nworie had a fitful night sleep.

When it was daylight, the village Doctor came again to Mr. Nworie's house with even stronger analgesic drugs. He was cautious when administering aspirin and opium. When he was done with the routine injections, he joined the on-going discussion in the house because Mr. Nworie's kinsmen had already assembled in the corridor expressing opinions and counter opinions on the issue at hand and about who was the best bone setter to be invited and to handle Mr. Nworie's fractured bones,. The oldest man among them asked the village Doctor about his view, on who to invite to handle the legs. The village Doctor emphasized the need for the family to make a choice. He was ano-dyne in nature. His independent opinion was clear and visionary. Mrs. Nworie was quickly invited to the meeting to choose a trustworthy bone setter without delay. She looked grieved as she talked. She went for a man from a neighboring community who resided more than 35 kilometers away. Two men among the kinsmen were chosen to fetch the bone setter with speed. They were Okezie and Nnamuchi. Having arrived at this stage, the village Doctor went off to attend to other patients. He promised to return soon.

Nshioke Nwokpolo had been a traditional bone setter for a long time. His popularity spread across villages, communities and cities because many people had often testified of his expertise in handling dislocations and fractures. The man's natural gift was made visible in the Ameyor village through an old woman known named Nwobushi. Nwobushi was returning from the farm one day, bearing a basket of cassava, when she fell on the village road and dislocated her left leg. Hence Nshioke was immediately invited and he pushed the bone back to its formal position. Within a short time, Nwobushi was healed by the magical massage, therefore; the rate at which Nwobushi was healed, thrilled Mrs. Nworie to go for Nshioke. She perceived him as the best bone setter in the territory. The rural bone setters were close to chiropractors but they were unschooled and did not handle serious bone diseases.

The two men who had went away to fetch Nshioke arrived at his house when he was about to leave. His old bicycle was already in front of his tiny cabin. They exchanged greetings. He did not quite know them nor from where they come from, but the other man (Nnamuchi) with a puzzled frown on his face knew them. He was the one that introduced them and shared their griefs. He pleaded with him to join them and go to the Ameyor village without delay. He smiled inwardly and agreed. That was his job! The man went into the cabin, had brief words with the wife and then took hold of the paraphernalia he needed for fractured legs. He climbed upon his bicycle, as did the messengers, because they came there riding a bicycle. They headed to the Ameyor village.

Before their arrival, the village Doctor was there checking blood pressures. Mr. Nworie's kinsmen were at the corridor waiting impatiently, while the crowd kept growing in the corridor. Some of the soft hearted villagers flinched at the sight of the accident victim and folded their arms. Nshioke need not be shown who the injured was in as much as Mr. Nworle's penetrating cries echoed through the village. The man greeted the kinsmen with a smile and trotted towards Mr. Nworie. Nshioke was really in an ebullient mood, he had a penetrating gaze when he looked on the injured and felt sorry for them. He consoled him. Nshioke's arrival helped ease the tension in the house. The village Doctor raised his head and looked at him, he waved at him nodding in appreciation. He too nodded in gesture.

Both Nshioke and the village Doctor were immediately invited to the kinsmen meeting to discuss how they would change the life of the man in whose house they were when the village Doctor finished attending him. They came and sat down among them. As in many societies, the Ameyor village had learnt over the years, they had an almost paternal sense of responsibilities for their indigenes and a constant awareness that everyone must play a part in decision-making to ensure that they stay united. To a large extent, they surrendered to the ineradicable of belonging to one another. However, the oldest man addressed Nshioke.

"Our hearts are filled with grief over the incident that has brought our brother to bear pain on the bed. The hearts of the children, the wife and hordes in this compound are broken. You have seen the victim. Are you very sure that you can treat him and make him walk again?"

"It's a pity and very painful that such a calamity befalls your beloved one. I can treat him and God willing, he shall walk again." A huge man spoke up from behind:

"You have had a long term reputation in your treatments of fracture and dislocation hence we are convinced without reservation that you are the best in the region. Please do not fail us. We do not want to waste time, contact us whenever you notice this case beyond you."

"It's true! Pride goes before a fall. It is important you get us aware of any impediment to his quick recovery" said the oldest man.

"I will do my best. Thanks for the privilege."

"May the gods bless your hand".

"I'm very grateful."

Nshioke mentioned some of the things he needed to be done for him for a start, Kai-Kai was one of them and this made the people to give him a plank stare. His demand of Kai-Kai to be on the table every day he comes came as a big surprise to the family. The village Doctor didn't request for such things. But they agreed to get the local hot drink for him, in order to attract efficient service delivery. The village Doctor assured them of his presence every day, until there is improvement in Mr. Nworie's situation. They thanked him for all his hard work and commitment. Due to the nature of his job, he went out. Nshioke first had a brief discussion with him. Nshioke himself turned to his bicycle and untied the black cotton bag. He made his way with the bag toward Mr. Nworie who layed flat with his face up. He applied a local black balm around the edge of the affected leg and began to press the bones to join each other again. Mr. Nworie shouted in agony, calling the ancestors to intervene in his situation. More than four people were holding him and they pressed him down on the bed so that he will not in anguish distort the best treatment. Mr. Nworie was a huge tall man hence to control him wasn't child's play. When Nshioke was done, he rubbed the balm over again and applied it bead-like, which he made with palm frond around the broken part to gird the separated bones together for growth. Mr. Nworie was indeed in great suffering. His wife was desperately busy as she served, provided and cared for those present. Nshioke executed his skills perfectly and was given palm wine since Kai-Kai was not available. He greeted them after and left Mr. Nworie in loving hands. It was only the left leg he attended to.

On the following day, he came again in the morning before sun set to treat the right leg, there were only a few people that were there. These helped in holding Mr. Nworie in a fixed position during the bone setting. Mr. Nworie's struggle to remove Nshioke's hand from his body due to pain, was useless. Nshioke's hands were firmly placed to the affected part as he massaged and pressed the broken bones in the traditional way. Mr. Nworie cried, cried and cried as the pains circulated his whole body. Nshioke finished and sat on the pavement drinking Kai-Kai when the village Doctor arrived for the morning treatments. Nshioke was a very slim man and yet he took a lot of alcohol after duty. He was becoming addicted with the local hot drink, which could be very dangerous to his health.

It was quite unfortunate that Nshioke treated Mr. Nworie for more than five months and there was no sign of improvement. He could only sit on the bed extended with help, which he started doing few days after the accident. A huge amount of money had been give Nshioke, yet the delivery was very poor. Mr. Nworie's family timely observed that waiting for Nshioke to make the injured man walk again could be derailed. They became tired of him. The family even began to make fresh plans for another bone setter to take over. With information that they got from concerned citizens, three women in Ebonyi State were reining in the bone setting skills. Mrs. Nworie sent for them from where they resided in their Ezilo community. A thorough arrangement was made for them in the first place, because they worked as a team. The family had already believed in them even when they had not seen them.

Upon the invitation, the three women arrived on that Orie market day to see the man who fell from the tall palm tree. Their presence led to a powerful sacrifice done in the compound. A local pure white fowl was indecently slaughtered, its blood was poured on the door and corridor leading to the room where Mr. Nworie stayed. There were other things the blood was used for, in order to quench the powerful evil forces that had become an obstacle to Mr. Nworie's speedy recovery; some of the feathers were well utilized. The fowl was later

41

roasted and the meat was used to prepare a porridge yam, which they ate. The three women were traditionalists and they were bared by the gods from certain foods and conducts. In fact, they adhered strictly to the warnings of the gods, those native practices which they believed in kept them safe from all danger and their hands were favored. Having completed the rituals, they got into a conversation with Mr. Nworie and his family. It was a well concluded meeting, both parties agreed on the terms and conditions that applied. Their discussion did not deteriorate into any argument hence the family admired their dogged determination to get it right. An enormous amount of money was accepted by both parties, payable installments, and the three of them while they may not be able to come at once, twice a week was agreed. Their takeover of Mr. Nworie's case, raised hope. Of course, Nshioke's contract was terminated immediately.

Mr. Nworie's was treated by the three women for more than four months, but he could neither stand nor walk. The family became exasperated. A lot of money had been spent, time wasted and proportional income no longer flowed into the family as usual. Mr. Nworie's improvement, which had been hoped for never came. Being that hope springs eternal, Mrs Nworie and two men began to visit shrines, idols and dibia for more spiritual insight into Mr. Nworie's recovery. A lot of sacrifices were finely recommended and they offered the sacrifices to the gods using fowl, goat, pigeon, dog and snail. There were other items presented to the gods on the village road in the midnight. One of the dibia they visited in his shrine asserted that there were spiritual forces blocking all the concerted efforts being made to make Mr. Nworie to rise and walk again. Hence he gave them two items that must be kept in the room where Mr. Nworie lived. The items consisted of a carved wood and a reddish tied wool.

While the village Doctor was assiduous to prevent necrosis in the man's body, by administering apposite drugs, he admonished Mr. Nworie's family to sell land for income and take the man to the National Orthopaedic Hospital in Enugu urban. He opined the need for an x-ray film to be taken of the two broken legs and to also consult an orthopaedic Doctor. His words were thrown away and they continued the traditional medicine. He did not quite grow tired or weary over the case despite the fact that his candid advice was not taken. Though the family would have loved to go to the hospital, there was just no money and they did not want to form a habit of land selling. Besides, they may not get a reasonable amount from any land sold anyway. Mr. Nworie had eight children, two of them were married and those ones came periodically to neaten the room where their father lied.

Sixteen months after the accident, Mr. Nworie was able to begin crawling out of the room. He had often craved desperately to get out of the room. The farthest place he could bravely crawl to was the corridor where he stayed and received frequent visitors. The man himself looked visibly pale. He was badly treated and it was obvious to him, he may not walk again. All of the treatments given to him ended up as a palliative measure, but he would have already gone to the dust if not for the frantic efforts of the village Doctor. One day, he summoned his relatives, kinsmen and family for a fair communication of his final decision. He didn't want to dissimulate. The whole family gathered together including the village Doctor and he began:

"I would like to express my sincere gratitude to all of you for the complete role each and every one of you have played to make me live and walk again. The signature of your efforts will remain indelible in my life. Thank you! My life is now marked with suffering, as it stands now, I may not be able to walk again. The bones have abruptly refused to join each other in the normal position." The sound of his voice sickened his wife. She started to sob expressly. They shouted at her to keep quiet. After all her husband was still alive. She listened and stopped sobbing because her pathetic tears had no solution for her husband's problem. The oldest man enjoined Mr. Nworie to complete his statements and he continued:

"My blood, bone and marrow and entire body are sick and tired of all the bone setters. Therefore, all the bone setters should go away from me, let me live as I seem destined. Gratitude's to the Dokinta, without you; I might not be talking by now." The wife was quick to

43

open her mouth: "I am crying because huge resources have been spent, and my husband is yet still on the bed. This is mysterious, but if this is the will of the gods, I will live to question it." Tears rolled down from her eyes. People sighed deeply and pitied the family. There was murmuring among them. The oldest man concurred:

"Mr Nworie, it is true we have stood by you all these lean months, and have made very positive contributions, but we are still ready to offer assistance when needed. We are your brothers, and will often do our best any time to help because the relative of the dead person is he who carries the corpse on the head."

On his own contribution, the village Doctor reminded them of the need for regular medical checkup and re-emphasized his previous suggestion to take Mr. Nworie to the city's hospital when money was available. This dismissed the crowd. It was succinctly clear that Mr. Nworie would remain crippled on the bed waiting for the day of his departure.

5

In the Village Church

Mrs. Nworie Edeani had a deep thought about herself and family over all the money spent on fetish things, which they believed could help her husband to be free from his situation. She realized those things were a wasted effort and she decided to begin to go to church. She finely communicated her intention to the husband and he could not opine on the issue. Her husband's silence was believed by her to be an outright acceptance and she made up her mind. The intelligent impulse of thought was translated into material rewards by the application of known principles. She went to the church early for the first time in January. She was in her flump cloth to seek the face of God on Sunday.

Within the church premises, the choir was practicing seriously with their song papers in their hands. A man was leading in the songs in the hall built with bamboo. Some men and church council members sat on the wood opposite them discussing while some others stood and laughed as they discussed on. People were trooping to the Catholic Church with chairs and bench because the church chairs were not enough. A group of boys were under the bean tree chatting away time. It was Sunday, so they all dressed well. Inside the church were many women and children, men and boys were few. They were praying the rosary waiting for the arrival of the Catholic priest. The church had only one closing door donated by a concerned citizen, but it was without paned window and the floor was still sand, yet it was perfectly roofed and plastered. In truth, the church lacked many things including no indigenes. The window space usually was where ventilation would come, but it was blocked for the reason of the boys that were presently sitting there.

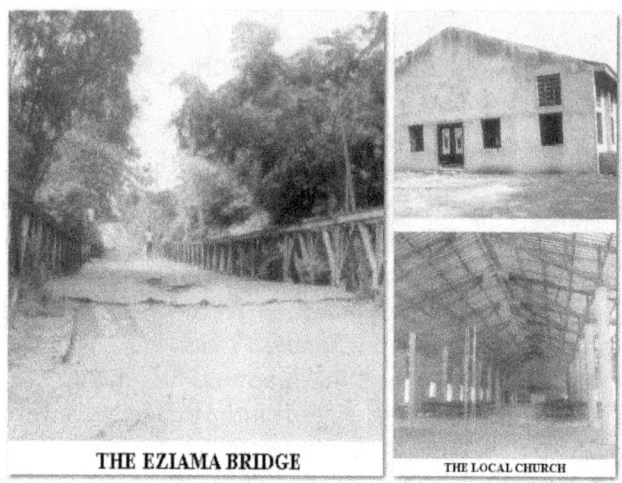

THE EZIAMA BRIDGE

THE LOCAL CHURCH

The village Doctor had always been socially positioned to the fore of the village. He was the church council vice and he was in the church with a Bible. The Catechist was on seat at the podium very close to the altar. People were going to him and leaving. The three entrances to the church had a bucket each and there were seeds inside them. It was expected of those who would take the Holy Communion to pick one. The church knew the number of all the seeds and would minus or plus when the time came to prepare the communion. The Catechist interrupted the rosary twice while making an announcement of great importance to the church. The rosy woman finished praying the rosary and more announcements were made as the altar boys got ready to serve in the mass.

At this stage, there was confusion in the church, because the priest was already 30 minutes late. The president of the Christian women organization began to sing to hold the church together. People were sighing and murmuring while more people left the church and stood in the compound to get fresh air. Being late was becoming part and parcel of the impenitent priest and he seemed not sound. He was flippant and he foisted his lateness to the church. The priest was saddled with the responsibilities to oversee three churches in different communities. He used to drive miles and miles of deserts to get to the two churches, because where he lived was the parish house and a church was there. He was tired of the bad rural roads. He made the church aware that if they want him to be punctual, they should make their roads more drivable and the bridge safer. The worn-out bridge was another huge problem for the community, it may collapse soon. There was no developmental project of the government in the whole area, so the indigenes must adapt to the condition, as it really takes time. The priest used to officiate in all of the three churches every Sunday.

Therefore, he was already 40 minutes late when he drove into the village church compound. He drove straight to the bamboo hall where he was fond of parking his car. The choir dismissed immediately and found their feet in the church; as soon as they settled down, they began to sing gloriously. All those in the compound rushed in to make them comfortable; two altar boys walked to the car and brought the suitcase, suntan and others. Pretty soon, the priest, and all those in uniform appeared on the altar as the congregation stood along singing to usher the priest in. Mrs. Nworie was all eyes as the day's Sunday mass began. She was completely bewildered.

However, the day's sermon came as a complete surprise to the villagers. The priest spoke on why people suffer. The three salient points were summarized and the villagers were perspicacious.

"It is comforting for us to know that God does not cause suffering. He is not responsible for the wars, the crimes, the oppression, or even the natural disasters that cause people to suffer. The Bible clearly states:

'The world is lying in the power of the wicked one.' (1 John 5:19) This world reflects the personality of the invisible spirit creature who is misleading the entire inhabited earth.' Satan is hateful, deceptive, and cruel. So the world, under his influence, is full of hatred, deceit and

47

cruelty. That is one reason why there is so much suffering. The second reason why there is so much suffering is that, mankind has been imperfect and sinful ever since the rebellion in the Garden of Eden. Sinful humans tend to struggle for dominance, and this results in wars, oppression, and suffering (Ecclesiastes 4:1) A third reason for suffering is 'time' and unforeseen occurrence.' (Ecclesiastes 9:11) In a world without God as protective Ruler, people may suffer because they happen to be in the wrong place at the wrong time. Church.' God has allowed Satan to show how he would rule mankind. God has also allowed humans to govern themselves under His guidance or Satan's influence (Revelation 22:11-12) church! God has not told us why he allowed suffering but I want you to know that He cares for you (1 Peter 5:7, Job 34:10)".

People were already shedding tears in the church, Mrs. Nworie was one of them. They thought they inherited suffering from birth. Mrs. Nworie believed she had been missing the word of God all those lean years. Because of the day's sermon, the church hated Satan. Therefore, the parish priest having ended the sermon, prayed and offertory was collected. He quickly blessed the communion and people lined up to receive, but something happened! The communion was not enough and many on the queue did not receive. There was murmuring in the church when the priest got back to the altar signaling the end of the day's Holy Communion. The communion was preselected according to the number given.

During the announcement time, the parish priest was the first to speak:

"Church! Obedience is better than sacrifice, for this reason, do not disobey even in the church. The seeds in the buckets are there for you to pick, if you have prepared yourselves to receive the Holy Communion according to the Catholic doctrine. Sacristy is not in this village church where some that are left over should be kept, that's why we produced the seeds, to know the number of people that will be receiving." The Catechist swiftly expounded the cause.

"Father! The mistake is not from the church. One hundred and ninety picked the seeds but the altar boy made a mistake and counted only ninety."

Murmuring went round the church. The priest was nearly red with anger but he controlled himself and began:

"Catechist! There are things people should not do for you. You are serving the public. You can only delegate duties to those who are capable otherwise, there will always be mistakes. By the way, where is the boy that counted "the seeds?"

The boy had already hidden himself at the local vestry where the priest dressed. His presence was required; the Catechist went in and brought him. He shuffled to the altar and the priest shouted:

"Church! Here is the boy that denied you Holy Communion!" The church was full of laughter. The village Doctor murmured something to the ear of the man sitting with him. Therefore, the priest cracked a joke with the church for a moment and then he continued:

"Today! We shall do a second collection because as previously announced, we shall do a new year for the Catechist. You know very well that it is at a time like this that we use to say 'well done' to the Catechist. Please dip your hand in the purse or pocket and support." He handed the microphone over to the church emcee and he began:

"Brethren! I went to the Catechist's house on the Christmas day hungry because I thought I would wine and dine with him, but Lo and behold there was not even a cup of rice in the pot. There was no food for the family let alone for visitors." The emcee always made people laugh. Some laughed scornfully while others pitied the Catechist. What the emcee said, motivated the church and second offertory was made. The Catechist was very gratitude to all of them. He made announcement for the weekly routine activities and the priest took over the microphone. He began again:

"Church! It is important you note that anything brought to the altar during offertory procession belongs to the priest – edible and none edible. Although, certain things I will not take but it is good you note this. If you want to donate anything to the church, inform the Catechist and space would be made available for you to do so." He dismissed the congregation. The church was well attended that day. The Catechist who had been very dutiful went home with the money handsomely contributed for him.

Mrs. Nworie learnt a lot in the church. Many women hugged her and appreciated her being in the church. The Christian women organization president made her aware she should start attending catechism because it is only when she is baptized that she can join organizations and enjoy certain privileges. She agreed to start catechism which was usually done in the evening. The church received her with open arms, and she was very happy. They assured her the priest would visit her husband, someday.

When she got home, she removed the charms in her house. She shared the story of the events that took place in the church to her dear husband, and how plans would be made soon for the priest to visit him. The man's mood oscillated between anger and elation. He believed in those charms but he also needed the presence of the parish priest.

Mrs. Nworie had demonstrated the attitude of hunters. However when hunters stay afar off and point at a certain bush, if there are no tigers there must be lions or both within its confine.

6

The Foreign Visitors

Many decades ago, the Ameyor village contributed largely in overseeing that Timothy Nnaji went to school to receive a good education due to his brightness and interest in education. He attended the elementary and secondary schools out of their pockets. He was as industrious as many of the other students and thereby elevated the name of the village school through his skills in the long jump, quiz competition, and in taking the first position in his class. There was no secondary school in the village when he was growing; hence the village unanimously sponsored his education in the township school. He continued to do well in class activities and in sports. He was notated by the state government during the inter-school competition due to the skill he demonstrated in quiz at the township school. Two students were chosen to represent the state at Lagos Nigeria, and he was one of them. Of course, he was very happy and they went along with all the officials concerned. At the Lagos Quiz Center, many states were represented. Enugu State performed remarkably well hence their students were given scholarships to study at the North Carolina University as soon as they completed the secondary school education. The Federal Government University Scholarship paved the way for someone from Ameyor village to go to the university out of the shores of Nigeria. So, when the two students completed their secondary school education, the federal government moved them to the U.S where they would begin schooling. Timothy chose to study medicine while Udoka decided for town planning. Timothy eventually became a pediatrician. He was well exposed to new and advanced methods in this particular field. During his school days, he enlightened his fellow international and American students on Nigeria's culture and values and he also got valuable information on American and other people's cultures in return, thereby, promoting world peace and understanding. He settled in North Carolina after his studies and rarely visited home.

One day, he remembered home and planned a visit. His friend Greg Hill was to accompany him, Greg Hill was American and functioned as a Chief Ophthalmologist. He was enthusiastic to see if it was true that Africans were like monkeys that live on trees, because that's what he had been told, as he had never been to Africa. On that good Nkwor market day, they came down to the Ameyor village bearing cartons of drugs, eye glasses, and medical equipment. Greg was all eyes to see the trees where the Africans lived in, but what he actually saw was that those who lived in the village, lived in cabins, houses built with dried muds having grass-attached roofs with earthen floors, while others lived in cement houses made with zinc. This clarified his perceptual orientation about the Africans. Of course, they came down with a van; the two with the driver.

Generally, the village was ruled by His Royal Majesty who was the custodian of culture and security. Any Government official or dignitary, who came to the village, would report first of all to the Igwe. The Igwe would then consent and disseminate information through his cabinet or council of elders to the other subordinates. That was exactly what Timothy and Greg did, and were well received. On the following day all the villagers assembled at the primary school field, which was the village recreation center to welcome the foreign visitors. Multitudes of people stood in awe of Greg. It was their first direct contact with a white man. This happened in the month of July, the specific month of the community festivals. Masquerades displayed various ingenuousness' including young women between the ages of 15-25 who displayed theirs as well. Usually this was when men found their wives. Craftsmen dominated this major source of sustainability and they displayed their hand works as well. A group of people were beating the drums and making music for the entire all. The man who was playing the flute, thrilled Greg to laughter as he drew close to him while in motion. Few of those who played with Timothy in his tender age, flocked around him, as he looked younger than they. They appreciated the need for good education. Greg and Timothy were well entertained by the people with their cultures. His Royal Majesty appealed to the villagers to avail themselves of the full range of medical treatments that were being brought to their door step by the foreign visitors. He let them know that from Monday, the medical Doctors would be in the primary school available for free health treatments and checkups. He dismissed the crowd latter.

The second part of call in the village by the foreign visitors was the village Doctor. They visited his chemist shop in mid-morning when there were no customers. He was there alone arranging order in the shop when the foreign visitors arrived. After a friendly greeting, Dr. Timothy opened the discussion thus;

"You have been working so hard in treating the entire village. You have accomplished this feat alone with just the little experience and knowledge you have acquired as a paramedic. What do you have to tell us about the people we have come to treat?"

"First of all, thank you for coming. Your visit is timely."

"Okay! "Said Timothy, Dr. Greg nodded in agreement.

"The villagers are negative toward health personnel. They tend to seek medical attention only in a terminal emergency. They patronize herbs, which have failed many. Again, they are very conscious of the fact that money is hard to obtain and that a small amount must be made to go a long way. Hence they are not always disposed to patronize improved health services."

"Why is that so?" Asked by Dr. Greg.

"It is so, because we don't have a government that cares for her citizenry. The government does not have any program for the entire community hence poverty has walloped many. Since the creation of the world, the people of this area has never experienced any form of government's presence. The primary school was built by the people and the government has only sent teachers. In summary, the people of this area have been essentially abandoned by various successive governments, domestic organizations and international nongovernmental organizations."

"Pathetic!" Dr. Greg intoned.

"Oh! Well! We do hope that the villagers will come for the free medication on Monday. Their presence will prove to us that they really need to take care of their health."

"Thank you once again for coming. Perhaps I can rest awhile."

"Tarry! Your presence is needed at the dispensary section from Monday when the general treatment begins."

"The honor is mine." The discussion ended and the visitors dispersed quickly.

Therefore, the village primary school was the only open place in the village granted for the foreign visitors to use as a hospital. Able - bodied boys were assembled, who were instrumental in putting the school in a hospital shape. Drip stands were made of wood and bamboo that utilized heavy rocks and iron to support them down. Chairs were carried from three miles under the instruction of His Royal Majesty. The man himself came around to see how the new temporal hospital was being built. The school tables were brought over. An electrician was hired and he electrified part of the school that had been demarcated. He affixed a light bulb when he tested the power generating plant that Dr. Timothy bought. All hands were on deck from Monday to serve the village well, including Greg who was with broom dusting down the cobwebs. His Royal Majesty, while on a fact finding mission, brought a jar of palm wine for them. At the end of the work, they gathered and drank the palm wine in plastic cups. Dr. Greg enjoyed the palm wine, for it was his first time drinking it and he drank with caution. Dr. Timothy gave out cash to the young boys for unwavering volunteerism. They were blissful for his boundless generosity and they went back to their pleasant homes, after sharing the money among them. On Sunday, the visitors went to the local church. Dr. Greg was sorrowful over the church situation but was impressed by the villager's efforts in going to church. More announcements were made calling on the villagers to come for free health services on Monday. The Catholic Priest thanked the visitors for having a commonsense of humanity. He made them understand that God is watching them and would definitely reward them appropriately.

Before 8 a.m. on Monday, the villagers had already begun to troop in towards the primary school with all kinds of ailments. At 9 a.m., Dr. Timothy, Dr. Greg, Miss Ijeoma, Mr. Onyebuchi and the village Doctor arrived. Before their arrival, somebody was writing down the villager's names and issuing cards sequentially. Their arrival historically signaled the beginning of a new dawn of humanitarian service for the entire community. Dr. Timothy had come to give back to the poor villagers, who had previously contributed immensely towards his worthy education. However, Miss Ijeoma served as an interpreter to Dr. Greg and the local people during his consultations. She also served as a messenger. Mr. Onyebuchi was the coordinator of the health service activities in entirety; he primarily controlled the crowd and disseminated information. The village Doctor was fully in charge of drugs and their administration, as prescribed. More than 200 villagers were present, and in great need of medical attention. The mammoth crowd initially terrified Dr. Greg. He called the village Doctor and when he came to him, he asked him:

"Everybody here needs medical care?"

"Yeah! Toil and malnutrition have played major roles in what you see. Free medical care has never been given to anybody in this area. This is first time in history to our generation."

"Okay! I can understand they like our presence."

"Yes! Some of them are beaming with smiles of appreciation. Many of them have never seen people such as you. Can you see how they admire you?"

Dr. Greg laughed and the village Doctor walked back to his duty post. The coordinator announced that all those with eye problems should Queue up along the line unto Dr. Greg, while others should join the other line. The villagers obeyed, especially those who could stand because the aged people occupied the available seats. As the treatments were about to commence, a man collapsed. The man himself looked pale and tattered. Some of the villagers gave a shout of outrage seeing the man in the mud prostrated. Without delay, Mr. Onyebuchi and another young man lifted him up quickly and carried him into the embellished ward. The two medical Doctors and the village Doctor surrounded him. Dr. Greg located the man's muscle wrist quickly and injected the syringe, which paved the way for the drip. Dr. Timothy was busy at the other hand checking B.P, and the sugar level. The pulse was busily disappearing while the sugar level read high. The village Doctor walked from the drug section to where they were, carrying the drugs and other things. There were various treatments available for the man's condition and he received them as given. Upon stabilizing the man they therefore turned to the crowd and the treatments began, while the village Doctor monitored him frequently to check and see if his condition had changed.

The eyes of His Royal Majesty was first to be checked by Dr. Greg. Igwe complained of itching eyes hence an effective eye drop was dropped in both eyes by the village Doctor. Dr. Greg gave him matching eyeglasses and asked him to return on Wednesday for a check-up. He also gave him an ointment peculiar to his eyes and he thanked him. Dr. Greg took great care and time in checking the people's eyes. Those who could read were given alphabets to recite, but those who could not read were shown objects and then urged to identify the objects having one eye closed, so Dr. Greg could determine their visions. Checking eyes and making the rigorous calculations consequentially was indeed a herculean task. Dr. Timothy was busily engaged with the villagers in conversation as he checked the B.P, sugar level, heart pump and others. He spoke the local dialect when he gave advice and prescribed from the drugs they had in store. Mrs. Odinaka, whose body was badly scarred by chicken pox asked him what she could do to evade the disease for the rest of her life. She didn't want to be forlorn again.

"Bathe three times a day; Keep your surroundings clean and consult a medical expert from time to time."

"You mean I should leave everything am doing and bath three times every day?"

"Yes! You should also have your clothes clean. I can understand that many of you don't take a bath for days. Therefore, be prepared to live hygienically conditioned."

"Hmm! I have never taken a bath three times a day. I will begin to practice it. Thank you Doctor."

"You are welcome."

She went back home well satisfied. The man who suddenly fainted and was under intensive care showed signs of recovery when the village Doctor checked in on him at noon, but he was still akinesic (unable to move much). The village Doctor quickly alerted Dr. Timothy and he came and applied more drugs. The man had skin lesions too.

Dr. Greg discovered that cataract was the major problem of the villagers that he had examined. He set aside Wednesday for the surgical removal. Twenty people whose bodies were fit for the operation were given tags and instructions about the surgery, many of them were given ointment prescribed by him via the village Doctor. The medical team really worked tirelessly before the clinic was closed at 4 p.m. to avoid undue stress. Those who were not treated were asked to come the following day. The man who collapsed was discharged and asked to come tomorrow because he was now ambulant. The ever busy village Doctor then went over his shop to receive his regular customers, as not all of the villagers saw the need for the free medical checkup. Dr. Timothy and Greg who had never done this kind of odd job before, went home to rest.

The clinic opened up on Tuesday and many villagers trooped in again. Dr. Timothy did a surgical operation that day, on a boy called Onyeka. Hernia had mesmerized this boy's life. Dr. Timothy postponed other treatments and consultations till Thursday before he proceeded with the emergency operation. The operation was very successful and the boy was hospitalized. However, the success of the hernia operation gave hope to the villagers who were afraid of going to the theatre. It would have been a total disaster if the boy had died during the operation. Dr. Timothy was indeed an experienced surgeon and he was also very excited. His adrenalin was really flowing.

On Wednesday, His Royal Majesty came to the clinic, as strongly advised. He informed Dr. Greg reliably that the eye drops he had given him were very effective, hence his eyes no long itched all within a few days of his attention. Dr. Greg was very happy for the strong testimony, and he urged him to take good care of the eyeglasses. His Royal Majesty, Igwe – Nnamani Nwokorie was very appreciative of the humanitarian services the medical team was rendering to the villagers. He reminded them that they would be remembered by what they had done for the community of people. He shook hands with all of them and praised them blindingly. When he was done chatting with the villagers too, he went back home with his usual entourage.

Meanwhile, fifteen people honored Dr. Greg's invitation for the cataract removal. Without mincing words, he made it clear to them that multitude people, who are blind today, had a cataract contributor but those ones either did not follow their Doctor's advice or had no one to detect their case, hence they villagers now had the opportunity to flee from blindness through this surgical removal. By this way, he prepared their hearts and minds because being ignorant of the law is not an excuse. Both Medical Doctors and the village Doctor were in the formal theater wearing uniform-blue. The patients were ushered in one by one as the minor operation commenced. Dr. Greg was a virtuoso in the field and he was as fast as was his expertise. The fifteen patients had their cataracts removed successfully. Dr. Timothy operated on four children, two hernia cases and two appendices. None of the patients died and it was evidence that their hands were blessed-albeit they operated under such a tight atmosphere. The village Doctor was all eyes to the operations through which he gained valuable experience whilst working with the medical Doctors. He was in the clinic all through the day, doing the village service. The visit of the two medical experts restored ailing sights and the life of many villagers. The villagers on their own part contributed to the good work being done for them, extending a lot of farm produce and palm wine to them in appreciation.

After a month in the village, Dr. Greg began to prepare to travel back to the United States. He had already finished treating most of the eye problems known. The entire village celebrated both Doctors for their achievements within the month. His Royal Majesty gave them chieftaincy titles; Dr. Greg was called Omemgbe Oji, while Timothy was named Ozo Igbondu. They were dressed in lion head clothes and red caps as title bearers. Ofo Igbo was given each of them. Dr. Greg extolled the villagers for their great hospitality towards them, while Dr. Timothy really appreciated his friend for adjusting his life style, and adapted to the local populace. He also extolled the virtues of simplicity seen in the village Doctor and his concern for the villagers. The village Doctor covertly informed Dr. Greg that the villagers would miss him, his smile and care. His Royal Majesty made him to understand he had become part of the community and can visit them whenever he is able. They wined and dined in the local way of life. Dr. Greg shook hands with many who cared. Before his departure, he extended an envelope of dollar to the village Doctor in support of his dedication in serving the village. He received it and the touch of it, gladdened his heart. The white envelop was fat. Dr. Greg hugged the medical team and he travelled back. The impeccable Doctor had imparted positively to the villagers. Dr. Timothy remained focused working together with the village Doctor and others. He still had three more weeks to stay.

It was in the village that Dr. Timothy first encountered a Kwashiorkor case since he became a pediatrician. He made the ailment open to the mother:

"Your daughter is suffering from Kwashiorkor Do you know?"

"Kwashiorkor? What is Kwashiorkor?"

"Kwashiorkor is a clinical syndrome where it was found that children who at weaning were put straight onto an almost protein-free local diet and showed a well-marked set of symptoms. The symptoms included lack of the black pigment melanin, which led to their skin color being a pale reddish-brown color rather than black, and their hair became pale and loose rather than black and tightly curled. Madam! Because of unbalanced diet, Kwashiorkor has set in this baby. I shall give you the food menu for children in this condition later."

"Thank you Doctor."

Dr. Timothy placed the kid on a strong vaccination and dietary regime. He took care of the child for a week in the village clinic and discharged her later due to the good changes in her body system becoming visible. He gave the mother the food menu and cash for the family up keep.

Due to the fact the villagers had no orientation on proper sanitary hygiene, dietary and or prompt action to a change in the body system, he held a-two day health seminar for them in the Catholic Church. In the seminar he also warned them of the dangers of streptococcus, the adverse effects of dilatation and curettage through the use of herbs and salt. He explained that bare feet are exposed to a number of pests ranging from the minor nuisance of jiggers to the serious infection of hook worms and guinea worms. The villagers were all happy for his informative concern for them. The seminar literally electrified them. The village Doctor assisted him strongly in the seminar's organization.

Three days before his departure from the village, the clinic was closed. It was already in September, and the school was now in its resumption period. The medical team vacated themselves for the pupils, who would resume the following week. They used two of those three days in visiting some of the sick ones at their respective homes. He handed the remaining drugs and medical equipment over to the village Doctor and warned:

"You are not qualified to treat all of the cases brought to you. Be cautious in your administration of drugs too, so as to avoid complications. Take good care of our people. I have known some of their major needs and will really do something further when I get back to the U.S."

"Thank you very much indeed! You healed wounds and restored hopes pleasantly. I will continue to do my best, in my own minor capacity."

Dr. Timothy laughed. He admired the village Doctor's humility and simplicity. He shared money with the medical team and they were very happy. They saw him off along with his own relatives and he travelled back to America. The foreign visitors' presence was indeed providential to the Ameyor village.

The village Doctor now had more equipment and vaccines to work with. The pamphlets and books that were given to him helped in serving the village better, as he read them.

"The glowing embers of fire placed in the palms of a child by a father do not burn the lad".

7

Salvation at Last

Dr. Timothy found out that he was the one who would alleviate the sufferings of the villagers and make their days better. Therefore, he did not waiver in his resolve to bring about a change to the villager's situation, neither folded his arms when he got back to North Carolina. He communicated his ideas to Dr. Greg, who also had the desire to help the Ameyor village, and they stood as one and as like minds and planned how the ideas could work. They embarked on programs that were intended to reach the general public in the U.S and beyond. They did this through Newspaper publications, radio and television and other media institutions. Of course, they shared their experiences in the Ameyor village when they were there on humanitarian service and presented some pictures which illustrated the full story. Yes! Dr. Timothy had made the general public aware of what it is actually like to live in that village. That quality health service was still a rare phenomenon in the area. Dr. Greg informed his fellow compatriots thoroughly that it is too complicated to leave the life of an entire village/community in the hand of a village Doctor. He described the village Doctor as a hardworking and dependable man, who had no proper education, but had the determination to make the village salubrious −albeit his hands were blessed and the people testified. This story captured the hearts and minds of people to donate. That's how they mobilized good resources for a proper health institution for the villagers. Americans were generous in nature. Dr. Greg made speeches in Texas, Florida and Arizona before curious donors. Dr. Timothy made speeches in Pennsylvania, New York, North Carolina and Oregon.

Within the interval of two years, Dr. Timothy and Dr. Greg returned to the Ameyor village with lots of packages. Dr. Timothy also returned with his family this time for them to know their route. Dr. Greg was the strong proponent of his friend's initiative towards the villagers. Their presence made the villagers delirious with delight.

History was made at the village square where the poor were helped and the scholarship foundation launched. Twenty one students benefited from the Ameyor scholarship initiative being launched, and enabled them to study in any field of whatever their endeavors turned out to be. Dozens of mosquitos' nets were freely distributed and their usage was taught. Thirty youth were selected for a youth empowerment training program and a specific amount was mapped out for them to start life after the skill acquisition training. His Royal Majesty had no car and was given one. The village Doctor was rewarded with a motorcycle to enable him run the village business. The fat envelope given to him by an American women who heard his story was extended to him. Inside the brown envelop was a letter, two photos, a complementary card and cash. Tears of joy ran down his cheek because he never expected such a kind gesture from a stranger. He was on top of the world. The high point of the event was the request made for land allocation for hospital establishment in the village. His Royal Majesty whose heart had been filled with joy wasted no time in offering the public land at the center of the community without a second thought. In a while, he became conscious of this haste and he asked the villagers if he had offered the land in error, but nobody objected to the noble ideal. Dr. Timothy's children looked at the villagers and smiled. They were probably enjoying the events. Mrs. Timothy shared cloths, food stuffs, and envelopes to the women. The villagers danced and danced the local dance. It was hilarious to see Dr. Greg dance. He would have been a good dancer, but he didn't practice evermore. His Royal Majesty announced that a committee would be constituted to work with Dr. Greg and Timothy who had come to make their life better. The villagers were very happy and they prayed for them. It was a successful event and they dispersed.

According to the lights of His Royal Majesty, a seven man committee was set up to genuinely work with the two tireless medical Doctors to successfully establish a hospital in the land. The village Doctor was among them. His Royal Majesty invited nine of them to his local palace, where he and the council of elders admonished them to work co-operatively and wisely in achieving that great mandate. He released a letter to them empowering them to go to the community land. He also made the committee understand that its main assignment among others was to direct and provide a level ground for the community development, and should not relent in getting back with the council of elders where necessary. The committee headed by the village Doctor promised to work harmoniously and diligently with the committee and also to report the council once a month. Two youths that were among the committee were expected to carry the village flag with others when the light faded from the elderly.

However, the committee took to the other side of the foreign visitors and the portion of land allocated for the new hospital was shown. They liked the land. It was sandy and well situated. Dr. Timothy told Greg that it was now palpable that the villagers were ready for change. He responded with an affirmative and they began to work harder in executing the village project. Having seen the land, a surveyor was immediately hired and he went ahead in measuring the land allocated, for the benefit of record. Two construction firms in the city were then contacted to submit proposals for the hospital project. They were shown the hospital's design. Dr. Timothy came with the architectural drawing of the hospital of their choice. The feature of the drawing gladdened the committee and stimulated the contracting firms. At last, the Marlum Construction Company won the contract to erect the hospital building. Half of the entire sum was paid and work began immediately. Dr. Timothy pleaded with the contractor to employ the villagers so that they could also benefit. The firm agreed, for their own security too and the security of their materials, even though they were assured of adequate security. So, very many villagers were employed, as laborers. The foundation laying ceremony by the community leader attracted large number of villagers. The hospital project was indeed a novelty to the villagers.

As work continued with speed, the villagers came there to take sight of the work and workers. Some came with bicycles, some by foot and some came barefooted, hot sand burned those one's feet. The laborers worked with haste because a specific amount was paid them every day for each completed work assignment, by the assistant finance manager of the company. However, the project kept growing and Dr. Greg began preparations to travel to the U.S to arrange for the hospital equipment, drugs and other needed things to be sent. Both medical Doctors teamed up and wrote down all of the requirements including a power generating plant. The village Doctor prepared a charming parcel, which Dr. Greg should extend to the woman who sent him a white envelope. When Dr. Greg finished these assignments he traveled back. Dr. Timothy and the committee frequented the project site to ensure the good deed was done as expected. The civil engineers were always there overseeing the work of the carpenters and masons. They worked at the site every day except on Sundays. The traditional rural visited the site once in a week to chat with the workers. The benevolent wine tappers brought wine for the worker's enjoyment, while some farmers extended yam to them. The yams were roasted and they were served as lunch. So, the villagers liked the work being done and they contributed their quota in support because; *"when people urinate together, their urine will foam together"*. It was a two story building project with wards and quarters.

On his own part, Dr. Greg a man of considerable brilliant, even as he worked in his office, mobilized more supports to equip the hospital when completed. Meanwhile he handed the village Doctor's parcel to Sharon and she was flattered. The parcel came as a big surprise to her in as much as she was not expecting anything in return. Contained within the parcel included the following items; a photo, a hand writing acknowledgement, a thank you letter, a local necklace, and a video DVD film which was shot in the village by Nollywood. The film was an authentic representation of the then Ameyor village. (Stronger than Pain). She demanded for the possibility of speaking on phone with the village Doctor, Dr. Greg promised to make the arrangement. Therefore, philanthropists from Arizona donated the most expensive hospital equipment, drugs were donated by those in New York while others donated cash. Some of the equipment and drugs not donated but useful, were bought. Sharon volunteered herself too, and joined Dr. Greg in pursuing the village course. When all of the hospital equipment was properly arranged and documented; it was shipped down to Nigeria. Dr. Greg was indeed an epitome of a humanitarian servant, the line of communication between him and Timothy did not break. Notwithstanding, there was an arrangement for Sharon and the village Doctor to speak for the first time. They spoke jubilantly. The village Doctor was on top of the world for speaking with a white woman in the first place. Sharon gradually began to develop interest in the village Doctor and she asked Dr. Greg when she could see him. He told her that it is a matter of time. She was curious to know more about the village Doctor and Dr. Greg explained further.

The hospital project was beautifully completed within a year – hence set to use when equipped. Its marvelous aesthetic beautification caught the eyes of the villagers, many of whom have never stopped visiting the place. However, when the ship-load from the U.S arrived the Apapa Warf in Lagos, Dr. Timothy travelled there to assist the agent in clearing. Due to the Nigeria's way of operating at the Warf, the goods took several weeks even when he had all the supporting documents as evidence. Dr. Timothy was really frustrated in the name of security checks but he remained focused and grittily determined. After passing through the rigorous processes, the hospital equipment was released to him. His equable temperament effectively contributed towards the release of the load. Having received the hospital materials, three trucks were then hired to completely convey them to the Ameyor village and it took just two days for them to get there, as it was a far distance to travel from western Nigeria to Eastern Nigeria.

Dr. Timothy, a man of the people, quickly communicated to Greg for him to be quick in coming down to Nigeria with those who would assist in the hospital's take off. Dr. Greg wanted to bring Sharon to head up the hospital administration but she was regrettably already on a contract. She would have used that opportunity to meet the village Doctor, so, she handed a briefcase to Dr. Greg for the village Doctor. Dr. Greg came down to the village with 5 Medical Doctors, a professional hospital manager, a pharmacist, two nurses, a lab scientist and lab technician. Each of these visitors were very excited to be in Africa. They entered the village and mingled with the villagers and they took camera shots. The villagers were happy too, though communication with some of them was very poor because, not all the villagers could speak in English. Nevertheless, the medical team worked together in the installation of machines, equipment, and in the arrangement the entire building to suit a hospital environment. A big power generator set was personally manned by the indigene that lived in the township – he was an expert in the field – so the hospital brought him home. Apartments of the health professionals were well furnished. Having accomplished the hospital master plan, the hospital began full operation. The medical team manned different sections of the hospital and had a keen interest to set standards. All of the villagers had access to free medical care, to a limit and free hospital cards were issued them within the week of the hospital inception. The first baby of the hospital was a boy and he was named after the great gynecologist who oversaw his delivery - Smart. This was done meanwhile before the hospital and obtained the life license. The hospital committee was registered and began to operate properly; Dr. Timothy and the committee registered it where necessary and obtained the life license. The hospital committee eventually became the hospital board, as allowed by the initiators of the hospital project. His Royal Majesty was the board chairman.

A week after the hospital started operating in favor of the villagers, it was officially declared open by the Health commissioner in the state, in a ceremony organized by the board. Official opening of the hospital attracted the state and Federal Ministries of Health, Red Cross, and Medical association of Nigeria, Radio Nigeria, Nigeria television Authority, the villagers and others. Dr. Timothy being the Chief Medical Director spoke at length concerning the hospital project and stressed the need for governments at all levels to visit communities, to identify their needs for appropriation, and implementations for comprehensive developments. Dr. Greg introduced the entire medical team and he promised as the deputy medical director, to have the hospital ready for 24/7 medical services.

He announced various vacant posts for employment of those qualified. His Royal Majesty who had been all along bearing with smiles, made the closing remarks. It was a well attended ceremony, full of colors.

As the Ameyor villager district hospital began to function effectively, more people were employed. The villagers had the highest rate of the employment ratio, and were posted to the various sections where their gainful services were needed. So, the media in its bridge building broadcasted the new revolutionary hospital to the nation. This attracted patients with different ailments from across the nation. On his own part, the village Doctor's name was posted at the large pharmacy where he worked with Pharm (George Earl). The presence of the professional foreigners contributed greatly to the large number of patients who frequented the hospital, as there was this belief in the foreigners that they had the key to science and technology. People began to set up shops and restaurants near the hospital vicinity, hence the village was gradually becoming famous.

Surprisingly, Sharon woods had been working hard beneath the carpet for the village Doctor's international recognition in Carolina. She believed that such a man, who thoroughly dedicated himself under rain, under the sun, day or night providing medical care to the entire village, deserved an excellence awareness. Americans, who had often rewarded good efforts and great ideas, bought the idea. They sent an invitation to the village Doctor. He travelled along with Dr. Timothy and Greg. Sharon was already at the airport to receive them. The village Doctor was amazed in seeing her, she beautifully engineered his presence. They couldn't stop chatting.

Therefore, the crowd gathered in the great hall where the village Doctor received a salubrious award and the crowd cheered. Several people made speeches during the award ceremony including Dr. Timothy and Greg. The Village Doctor used that opportunity to convey the good will message of the Ameyor village for the supports rendered causing the rural hospital establishment in his vicinity.

He also said:

"When entering my shop in the Ameyor village, I experienced that old excitement that still made me feel slightly sick and weak at the knees every time. I wondered how on earth I would leave my people and go on holiday; I found in my people, a new part of myself that I have to take care of. This self-discovery led me to the helm of my people's health needs, day and night. Nearly always I've expressed the wish that somehow the government and people, who have love for humanity, can come to the aid of my people. The United States has been devoted to just this cause. You have extended a protective umbrella over these forgotten villagers with the very best medical protection available.

You have judged well my merit of this award. It is crucial. Thank you!"

EPILOGUE

If the world should close their eyes and think that every community of people both in the rural and urban in African, have health centers or hospitals then the world have not been told the truth. It matters much that nations and the world at large ensure that every community has a well equipped health center or hospital available to attend to their needs. Again, rural and urban health services should be affordable at all times and health workers should live up to their calling to avoid more damage to humanity.

Your contributions to sustain someone's life would never be in vain.

Watch This Space – African Child's Dilemma.

ABOUT THE AUTHOR

Mr. Nwani Christian is from Enugu State Nigeria. He is an Evangelist, a Youth leader and a Researcher. This is his second book.

His first book is called "The Crys of the Ambitious Village Boy"

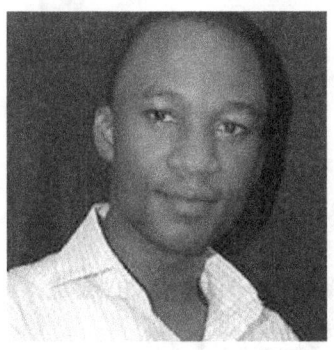

To write to the author

Both the author and publisher appreciate hearing from you.

Please write to the author:

villageboy489@gmail.com

Resources

Other Books By Nwani Chistian

The Crys of the Ambitious Village Boy

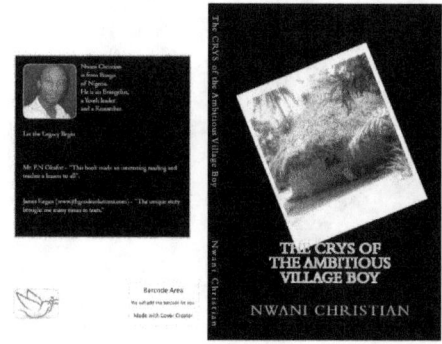

Other books of Interest:

-Frameworks: The Price of Delusion

-Effective Entrepreneurial Action

Find links to books and authors at - www.jrbgoodesolutions.com

The Village Doctor

www.ingramcontent.com/pod-product-compliance
Lightning Source LLC
Chambersburg PA
CBHW070932180526
45168CB00003B/1043